DO YOU KNOW THE REAL YOU?

A LIFE HACKER'S GUIDE TO PERSONAL GROWTH, DIET, AUTOIMMUNITY, EXERCISE, LOOKS MAXING, ATTRACTION SCIENCE, AND DATING

Wayne Vogel

DO YOU KNOW THE REAL YOU?

A LIFE HACKER'S GUIDE TO PERSONAL GROWTH, DIET, AUTOIMMUNITY, EXERCISE, LOOKS MAXING, ATTRACTION SCIENCE, AND DATING

BY

Wayne Vogel

Disclaimer

DISCLAIMER: THE INFORMATION CONTAINED WITHIN THIS BOOK IS FOR EDUCATIONAL PURPOSES ONLY AND IS NOT INTENDED TO BE A SUBSTITUTE FOR MEDICAL/CLINICAL CARE OR LEGAL ADVICE. PLEASE CONSULT A HEALTHCARE PROVIDER OR LICENSED ATTORNEY FOR GUIDANCE SPECIFIC TO YOUR CASE OR SITUATION. THIS BOOK DISCUSSES DIET, MENTAL HEALTH, AND LEGAL ISSUES IN GENERAL AND IS NOT INTENDED TO DIAGNOSE SPECIFIC CONDITIONS OR ADDRESS LEGAL ISSUES IN ANY WAY. USE THIS INFORMATION AT YOUR OWN RISK.

Dedication

This book is dedicated to: My Mom

Watching you struggle through all of your health issues and your pharmaceutically induced kidney failure has given me the strength to tackle all of my health issues and become the man I am today. You've been gone six years this year—crazy. I know that if you saw me today, you'd hardly believe it. I am sharing parts of our story, in your honor, to help others. I love you and miss you so much! Thank you so much for everything you did for me, Kevin, and your grandkiddos. I can only hope I am making you proud.

TABLE OF CONTENTS

Disclaimer iii

Dedication iv

Introduction 1

Chapter One: In Order to Know, There Must Be Change 5

Chapter Two: Dare to Compare 10

Chapter Three: The Impact of What You Eat 15

Chapter Four: Addition by Subtraction 20

Chapter Five: Margaritaville Part 1 – Sugar and Salt 26

Chapter Six: Margaritaville Part 2 – Alcohol and Substances 34

Chapter Seven: Autoimmunity 39

Chapter Eight: Getting Real About Doctors and Pharmaceuticals 46

Chapter Nine: Face Facts – The Science of Physical Attraction 52

Chapter Ten: Story of a Sloped-Chined, Crooked Jaw 57

Chapter Eleven: Through the Cracks, Facial Looks Maxing Process 68

Chapter Twelve: My Rant on Dating and More Attraction Science 75

Chapter Thirteen: Beneath the Surface 90

Chapter Fourteen: The Reality of Glowing Up 96

Epilogue 100

Bibliography 103

Introduction

Do you? If you think you know the real you, that makes sense. I thought I did. For years, I thought I was as good as I was going to get and that everything going downhill was normal when I started to age. Cramped-up muscles, fatigue, random issues, and declining looks just come with the territory, right? Wrong. I look and feel better now at 43 years old than I ever did at 33. What's better is that I was able to accomplish this feat without the inception of any pharmaceuticals or surgery. When googling one of my conditions for this research, Google claimed it was impossible to address without surgery. I am documenting that wild journey and much more here to help you.

If you have experienced health issues, I am truly sorry for what you have been through. I can also relate. Health issues and disease have ripped my family apart. By the time I hit my mid-thirties, I had lost both of my parents to terminal disease. The director at the funeral home told my younger brother and me that we were the youngest people he had ever seen with that burden. Even though I know some kids have it far worse, that perspective was still hard to swallow.

I did everything I could to help, including donating a kidney to my mom in April of 2010. However, shortly after doing so, I received the oh-so-joyous burden of being diagnosed with stage 3 chronic kidney disease myself. No good deed…On top of that, in 2015, right after my divorce, I was also diagnosed with a rare facial/cranial disorder. Then, in 2020, I began experiencing autoimmune issues. After feeling sorry for myself for a short while, I decided to start to address these issues without much luck. Experiencing my health issues seemed to be my genetic fate, if you will. As you can imagine, when I eventually started dating while all this was happening, I didn't have much luck there either. That's actually putting it mildly. Like many who attempt to date online, I experienced rejection on a vast scale.

Then, in late 2021, I experienced an awful heartbreak. That heartbreak and the subsequent healing process inspired me to write my first book, *From Brokenhearted to Brave*. The result was simple. Instead of trying to give all this love I claimed to have for a woman I was waiting to show up, I decided to turn it around on myself. What soon followed was the self-improvement journey of a lifetime. I became obsessed with improving myself and my health. And since my mom's kidney disease was caused by a pharmaceutical drug created by a company that eventually went bankrupt due to the class action lawsuits against it, I was hellbent on doing so all naturally.

Within this book, you will find some of the most well-researched and documented methodologies for addressing issues we eventually all face as humans. Succinctly put, the information recorded in this book helped me pull my life out of the doldrums of despair. I have studied optimization techniques now for years, using myself as the host. In doing so, I discovered who the real me really was. Genetics are a form of wealth; you need to optimize yours and polish your diamond to see what you really have.

As part of my journey, I have listened to countless advice from YouTube and podcasts and read dozens of books. I am going to state what many would agree to be obvious: Most information people spew in these areas is trash. Many of the books I read were garbage. So much of the advice doesn't work or is inept. There are only four books I will even reference or cite and only two I'd actually recommend most people read. As such, part of my perspective is also personal-medical-history-based and somewhat anecdotal. As part of this book, I will provide the value of skipping the endless minutiae and give you actionable steps that will lead to results the quickest. As you can tell, I hated stepping in all of the bullshit I found. There will also be summaries at the end of most chapters for quick re-referencing.

But what makes the advice in this book truly unique is the intertwinement of various strategies utilized to develop paradoxical solutions. Also, if you don't want to be a gym rat and largely enjoy being sedentary like me to achieve results, this is your jam. Being the IT nerd I was as a kid evolved into becoming a life-hacker—which has, in turn, made me a bit of a health scientist. I am not a doctor, but my childhood best friend I grew up with is, and he informed me that this is effectively what scientists do. Don't worry, though. Nearly all the advice I reference is from expert doctors in their various fields. Until we get to looks maxing…then I become the expert!

So, armed with this context in mind, we will journey together into all the information that will unquestionably better your life and, most importantly, help you get to know the real you. I cannot wait to see what you think!

Chapter One: In Order to Know, There Must Be Change

"Courage is being scared to death and saddling up anyway." – John Wayne[1]

Don't worry—this book does not lead off every chapter with a trendy and somewhat irrelevant quote from some random celebrity. I just like this quote for this chapter because change, like most celebrities, is scary. Not changing is pretty easy; it only requires one thing: inaction. If you're looking to discover the wonders of your true self, though, it's a pretty shitty thing to do. Comfort always comes with its costs.

When having a gander at the seven deadly sins the other day, I didn't know what 'sloth' was. Come to find out, it means laziness. I don't know about you, but I kind of love being lazy. It used to be my thing. Thinking about how far I had to go and how much I had to do was already exhausting enough. But, after studying change for my business book ventures, I realized I had the concept of change all wrong. When I realized the truth of how change worked, it then became quite motivating.

When preparing for this book, I knew I needed to lead with this topic. With this being the fourth book I've now written, this is the only one subject I have covered in each of them. Change, on the surface, is hard. There are also books I read on the topics of motivation, habit creation, and the like. None of them, however, addressed the animal in the room: expectations. Now that I've been on the other side of motivation for a few years, I realize that bullshit expectations kept me from even starting. The problem is, it's the uphill climbs that are the ones worth the view.

When I started tackling my jaw problem in 2021, this was exactly the one thing I chose to let go of. I told myself that no matter what, I was going to stick to doing one specific exercise a day and commit to it for a whole month. After day one, nothing. Day two, same thing. One-week, same story. But, one month? I noticed an ever-so-*slight* change. It's all the evidence I needed to keep going. And thank God I did! Fast forward to 2025, and I have accomplished the unimaginable. Now, just imagine if you could tackle your problems in the same way.

The fact is, meaningful change is a slow grind—a small, incremental, and iterative process. A great analogy is like travelling down a switchback road. When you're driving on one with a bunch of hairpin turns, you have to move slowly to ensure you stay on it. Change is the same way. It's tricky, too, because only we ourselves have the ability to change. We ultimately control it. Now, knowing that results take time became beyond motivating for me. I was able to let go of that picture of perfection I held in my head for so long and let go of that need to achieve it right away or as quickly as possible. The need to be perfect causes inaction; it's a fear that no matter how hard we try, we can't be as good as someone else.

The concept of perfection is the issue, not the concept of comparison, which we will discuss in the next chapter.

Small changes help you build up to larger ones, too. Changes are interconnected and have cross-functional impacts on improvements. Growth, like many things in life, also requires change. I'm going to share a secret with you, an epiphany I wish I had known long ago. If you want to earn love and respect, you must display evidence of love for yourself before someone else of value will believe it. Love for yourself is tricky; oftentimes, it's disguised as discipline, patience, and persistence through varying degrees of struggle.

IN SUMMARY:

- Change takes time, so commit to loving yourself through the process. Move your energy mostly away from the result and instead towards the effort.

- The solution for laziness is diligence when you don't feel like you should keep going. The solution for anger at the lack of results is patience.

- Results take time, but with the proper expectations, they will always follow. They may not always be what you want the first few times, but results are always the conclusion.

- Learn to measure yourself objectively, and make enhancements to your protocols based on those assessments.

- When starting out with these ventures, know that resistance is your compass. If you are actively avoiding something you know is good for you, chances are that is a great sign that it's exactly what you should be doing to better your future.

- Action will always make you feel better. Pay attention to your moods as a result. And, it's a guarantee you will always learn from it, too.

Since we started the chapter with a quote, let's end on one too:

"The measure of intelligence is the ability to change." – Albert Einstein[2]

Let's be intelligent and change over to the next chapter, shall we?

Chapter Two: Dare to Compare

I know what you might be thinking, "But Wayne, don't you hear 'comparison is the thief of joy' all the time?" And that would be correct—you do. One of my favorite things in life is to be correctly contrarian. Comparison is like most things: too much of it, and it's not good for you. But if you throw out comparison altogether, you could really be missing out. Utilizing comparison for valuable reasons like determining the goals you want to achieve is personally my main reason. Being a contrarian here can also help you determine what your strengths are, too. As you'll witness by my next story and analogy, we often do not get the full picture of comparison correct either.

In August of 2019, after a long summer day of jeeping in Estes Park, my children and I went back to a friend's house for some dinner. When we arrived, my friend had a neighbor there who swung by with…his brand-new special edition Lamborghini Huracán. The estimated retail value is right around $300,000. For some inspiration to write this chapter, I went back and looked at the videos of my kids revving the engine. My son was 12 then, so he got a big kick out of it! The Lambo owner was a surgeon about 15 years older than me. I personally don't have money like this, but I still thought it'd be really cool to own one someday, obviously. And given that he was around with it and offered me a ride, I had to accept.

While cruising around, I began to ask him some questions—questions around ownership he said nobody had asked him before. Having a Lambo seems great on the surface, but I wondered what it was actually like. I asked him how much the car insurance was…It was every bit of another mortgage! I asked him about the maintenance costs and frequency, and again, I couldn't believe the answer. It was also a track car, so he had a custom truck trailer to haul it to events—even more costs. Then, he went on to explain some of the hassles of owning it. Getting it serviced was a pain. Its rarity breeds inconveniences you don't think about. I could go on, but I think you see my point. The experience on the surface did not match its actuality. Right there, I was able to kill any 'FOMO' (fear of missing out) of ever owning one.

Before I started my self-improvement journey, my targets for my physical appearance were fairly simple.

1) To look like someone from the 1950s body-wise. Thin, fit, and nothing over the top.

2) To have a jawline like Justin Bieber in the 'What Do You Mean?' music video.

You might laugh at that last one, and it's totally allowed. I look back and find it comedic too at that video living rent-free in my head for so long as 'cool.' There was good reason for that target, though, based on my dental history. If I hadn't compared myself to these people, I would have never had a vision for these targets. And even though I still might not look as good as Justin Bieber, the results I have been able to achieve baffled both my doctors and my orthodontist/TMJ specialist.

You're probably wondering why I am telling you all of this. The answer is twofold.

1) I want you to have specific targets in mind for your personal crafting, no matter how big or small they may seem. Success isn't found in achieving the exact comparison itself, just the amount of progress you make.

2) You will always be met with some measure of failure and resistance in the process.

The latter point is key. Failure to achieve progress with these comparisons is also part of the learning process. The amount of herald greats throughout history who talk about how much they've failed is astonishing. John Quincy Adams, Albert Einstein, Abraham Lincoln, Bruce Lee, Winston Churchill, and Thomas Edison *all* have quotes on failure. Like them, I have now realized there are always answers in losing. It still doesn't make losing desirable. It just makes it okay and acceptable.

The last point I'll make comes from the great late Kobe Bryant.

"Greatness is in infinite growth." – Kobe Bryant[3]

Ain't that right? This is also difficult as a lifelong Denver Nuggets fan to quote the famous Nugget killer

---

himself. Don't tell anyone I grew up with, but despite that fact, I actually really look up to him. The secret in this quote—and what has delivered some of my most important strides in my journey—is continuing to grow. Constant tweaking and minute changes can help make the largest of strides. Looking back at my journey, there were many times when a minor change or small detail made all the difference.

IN SUMMARY:

- Some comparison is healthy and useful. Remember to consider all factors when comparing what others have, too. Remember to be grateful for not having the problems that come with what you don't have, as well.

- Going after what you want and making progress makes accepting what genetic gifts you don't have loads easier. It's all about being the best you can be.

- Expect some failure, and then use it to optimize your process. You are unique to everyone; therefore, your journey will be, too.

- Never be afraid to experiment. See what works. See what doesn't. Test constantly. It's all a part of the journey.

Comparing the importance of this chapter to some of the others seems unfair. However, this chapter always needed to be included. It might even end up being some readers' favorite one! Regardless, I am grateful you're on this journey. Buckle up because now we are getting into the main course of the content! I can't wait to take a bite out of this next chapter. Dad puns for the win.

Chapter Three: The Impact of What You Eat

Don't worry again. This chapter is not a placeholder for me to tell you to follow some ridiculous fad diet or give you the reasons why I think my personal diet is best. It is, however, a placeholder to give you some data on diet versus exercise, how to target problematic deficiencies in your diet, and help you take the most foundational steps in your health improvement journey. Diet is just that, the foundation—the foundation of your health. Get it right, and life can be a delight. Get it wrong, and you'll be singing a sad song. There's the poet coming out in me again, but I digress. Succinctly put, the right diet can and will help curb the need for excessive exercise for weight balance. I am living proof. I guess that age-old adage 'you are what you eat' wasn't so far off. However, I still hate that phrase. Let's get into the research of why the impact of what you eat is king.

According to just about every source on Google and AI search results, diet is around 70 to 80% of overall health and weight management.[4] I personally believe it's higher, closer to 90%. What you do with that 10 to 20% of exercise is also key, though, and not what you think. I will address it briefly in this chapter, but much more on looks maxing later in the book. Based on this data, diet is overwhelmingly the key. It's the key to balancing your micronutrient and hormone levels. What are micronutrients, you might ask? They are simply the current levels of vitamins and minerals in your body. They fluctuate for various reasons, much of which we will cover in the following chapters. If you can largely manage them without much—if any—supplementation, life becomes a joy. You cannot put a price on feeling healthy. Therefore, prioritizing these levels is the most important way to manage your diet. I will discuss the most effective way to do this in the chapter summary to help you create a personalized plan.

The problem with so much of the diet advice these days is that it simply does not address this crucial level of granularity. In fact, it's not possible to without *individualized* scientific evidence to support their claims. Overgeneralized claims that certain foods over others cause or prevent conditions like cancer do not include more detailed factors like a person's epigenetics and family health history. Partner that with the fact that several of these diets also actively cause various micronutrient deficiencies without supplementation, you have a recipe for disaster. It's no wonder why overgeneralizing is one of the lynchpins of idiocy.

Diets should also only be considered general guidelines for most days. Stressing out about what foods you eat constantly is counterproductive at best, unless you have a dangerous allergy, of course. I also cosign to and practice the once or twice-a-week cheat day recommendation to reward a good job of sticking to your diet most days (once-a-week is preferred, but twice-a-week needs to be spread out and never with back-to-back days). If you are tasked with regularly avoiding certain foods as a genetic recommendation, you still need to ensure you are consuming them from time to time to ensure you do not develop an allergy to them. If you are out to dinner periodically, stressing about ingredients that aren't genuine allergies is going too far. However, what we buy from the grocery store matters. All the days we eat at home add up, and that's where the true progress is made.

As an example and testimony to these points, I will share bits of my personal story. After trying multiple fad diets over the years without longer-term health benefits, I decided to engage a health clinic to measure my micronutrient and hormone levels. The results shocked me. I was diagnosed with one of the rarer forms of a MTHFR gene mutation. Even though it sounds scary, MTHFR gene mutations are very common, with around 60 to 70% of the population having at least one variant.[5] This gene affects the body's ability to process folate and, therefore, impedes methylation. Without going too far down the rabbit hole of methylation, let's just say it's very important to your health. It helps with DNA repair, immune response, hormone production, neurotransmitter production, energy production, detoxification, and inflammation. That's a lot. As you can imagine, once I addressed this via my diet, it was a game-changer. I will touch on these personal impacts later as it relates to some other health conditions as well.

IN SUMMARY:

- Diet is adopted by several health care providers as more important than exercise for weight control and general health.

- Get into a telehealth clinic like Marek Health ASAP for personalized health optimization services. They pull far more lab data than a PCP/General Medicine doctor can and still accept HSA dollars for their services.

- The data in your lab markers gives you the power to craft an individualized diet optimal for your personal specifications. Address any micronutrient deficiencies via your diet by googling what foods are high in those areas.

- Make occasional generalized exercise fun. Exercise when you can and combine it with other things you want to experience (sightseeing, etc.), but typically prioritize diet over exercise at all costs.

- Adopt a 'follow the sun' diet mentality. Only eat foods that are in season, less fats in the winter, more fats in the summer, etc. Try not to eat the same foods every day, and mix them up routinely. Try new things periodically.

Several times at the end of the chapters in my books, I like to tell a dad joke. Here's what I came up for this chapter: Why did the chicken cross the road? Answer: To show the vegans and vegetarians on the other side what they're missing! I'm sorry if you currently follow one of those diets, but I couldn't resist. Let's shake our tailfeathers right into the next chapter.

Chapter Four: Addition by Subtraction

If we were talking about arithmetic, this statement wouldn't make much sense. But since we are talking about self-improvement and health in general, it makes perfect sense. Quite a bit of the information covered in this chapter isn't necessarily something you see results from initially. Sometimes in life, it's all about prevention. As I have found with my constant tinkering, every so often the products or supplements we use cause the issues we have, especially after cleaning up our diets. Quite a few companies you wouldn't suspect don't want to solve your issues; they want to manage as many symptoms as possible to collect your money with their products. In my humble opinion, there's a much better way. Let's get into all of the points where adding by subtracting helps you avoid this sub-optimalization.

I will speak about personal experience soon, but I wanted to kick this topic off by bringing in quotes from an expert toxicologist. In researching this topic, I already knew I'd find lots of expert info to pull from. Most of us are aware of avoiding certain products for one reason or another. However, the scale is what's shocking. Quotes from a leading toxicologist named Dr. Yvonne Burkart regarding shampoos and deodorants confirm what I suspected: "For the most part, if you grab a product off of a store shelf, nine times out of ten there are chemicals of concern in them,"[6] and "All

---

antiperspirants contain aluminum salts, and aluminum itself acts like an estrogen in the body and increases the risk of breast cancer in young girls,"[7] just to name a few. Other recommendations to avoid indirect sources of concern she references are "Cookware and utensils can cause cancer—replace your cookware with PFAS- PTFE- PFOA- PFOS-free cookware."[8]

I realize that most of these statements seem kind of conspiracy theory-esque on the surface. But in my own experiences, some of them have definitely rung true. On my commute to work when I was younger, I would listen to a radio show called 'Mike & Mike in the Morning' on ESPN radio. One of the Mikes would always swear by washing his hair once a week, claiming it kept the natural oils in and made it look the way it did. He definitely had nice hair. Despite my initial judgment of thinking this was kind of gross, I decided to give it a try. Before I reveal the results, I will add in a bit of comedic context. I never used to have nice hair. Most of the time, it looked like I stuck a fork in a light socket. It was always standing on edge. I could never get it to lie flat like the other kids' hair.

Enter Mike's process. I started simply soaking my hair in the shower water most days instead of using shampoo. The results were baffling. All of the results these products claimed, 'shiny, healthy-looking hair,' for example, arrived when I stopped using their product. Strange, right? I have also talked to other men on this topic. Recently, at a golf tournament, I met a friend of a friend who explained that not using shampoo or other products on his hair is how he managed to keep it. He had two older full-blooded brothers who were both bald by his age. He decided not to use these products on his hair at all, and here he is today, with a full head of hair. Coincidence? I personally think not…But you are certainly entitled to your own opinion.

This concept also applies to 'standard' food additives. GMO or genetically modified foods like 'maltodextrin' can increase risks of various illnesses. These risks include:[9]

- **Allergic Reactions:** There is a small risk that GMO foods can trigger an allergic reaction if the genetic change produces an allergen.
- **Cancer:** Some concerns exist about the potential impact of GMOs on cancer risk.
- **Antibacterial Resistance:** GMOs may transfer antibiotic-resistant genes to gut flora.
- **Changes in Human DNA:** The impact of GMOs on human DNA is still being studied.
- **Toxicity for Body Organs:** Research is ongoing to understand any potential toxicity of GMOs.

I will never understand how these foods are allowed by certain drug and food administrations. Look out for strange ingredients when shopping for your next grocery cart full of food. You might just be shocked at what you see.

I've even experienced similar results with nutrient supplementation. To increase my blood flow some years ago, I began to incorporate an all-natural pine bark extract supplement, which claimed to increase athletic performance and even enhance mental cognition by 15%. Then, about three months after incorporating this supplement into my daily routine, I suddenly began experiencing debilitating ocular migraines, temporarily causing me to go fully blind for a period of 30 to 45 minutes at a time. Needless to say, it was terrifying. After several doctor's visits with no causation in sight (no pun intended), I decided to extract this supplement from my routine (the pun was intended there). The result? I have never had an ocular migraine since. For me, this was definitely *not* a coincidence.

I think you see my point here. Many times in life, things you think of as good can begin to become bad. It's not always just about food, either. Opening your mind to the possibilities of this can become a game-changer for your personal protocol. Especially as I have started to age, these considerations have saved me immeasurable angst in dealing with and managing my health issues. Understanding that every product you put on your skin or in your body can have unintended impacts is profound. Please always think twice before incorporating the next hot supplement or hygiene product into your protocol. And the issues you are experiencing are likely not from what you think.

IN SUMMARY:

- Genetically honed and tailored diets reduce the need for hygiene products and supplementation. As a general rule, try to eat organic, simple, and whole foods as much as possible. This is more important with meats than produce, as most produce can never really be considered organic due to some of the grow processes.

- Limit all of the hygiene products you use in general, and search for all-natural ingredients in the ones you use, including soaps. As a general rule, keep products as far away from your head, hair, and face as much as you can.

- Beware of the risks of over-supplementation, even with standard vitamins. Sometimes, too much of a good thing can quickly turn into a detriment.

I hope by now you are beginning to see some of the ways we can analyze our own decisions and correlate them to the problems we encounter with our health. It's crazy, to say the least. Crazier than a Margaritaville party on a random tropical island during spring break? Maybe not. But, the information in the next few chapters will have you further pondering our nutrition and how we also choose to party! Let's get even more real in the next mini-series.

Chapter Five: Margaritaville Part 1 – Sugar and Salt

You might wonder why I decided to dedicate an entire chapter to these two. It's a good question. It may be surprising, but the balancing of these two has helped me solve problems in my life that I thought were unsolvable. You see, many people—and even medical advice—leave out their presence in the process of hydration. Understanding the truth behind it, instead of the age-old adage of "drink more water," has massive health benefits, especially for your skin. Sugar and salt, specifically glucose and sodium, play crucial roles in hydration by aiding in the absorption and retention of water in the body. Yet, when you view most advice on how to improve the look of your skin, they are never discussed. Both are even villainized routinely, so let's determine which one actually deserves the criticism and which one can solve many issues you wouldn't think of, shall we?

Let's first start with how glucose and sodium contribute to hydration:[10]

- **Sodium (Salt):**
  Sodium is an electrolyte that helps regulate fluid balance and is essential for the body to absorb water. It helps maintain the right balance of fluids inside and outside the cells.

- **Glucose (Sugar):**
  Glucose, a type of sugar, is transported into cells along with sodium and water, helping them absorb fluids more effectively. It is a primary energy source for cells and plays a vital role in transporting water and sodium across cell membranes.

- Essentially, glucose and sodium work together to create an environment that encourages the absorption and retention of water. Sodium helps draw water into the bloodstream, while glucose facilitates the transport of sodium and water across cell membranes. This synergistic interaction is essential for maintaining proper hydration and electrolyte balance.

Here's the typical recommendation for hydration: "For a standard glass of water, a typical amount of salt and glucose to add for rehydration purposes would be around 1/4 teaspoon of salt (or approximately 1 gram) and 1 teaspoon of sugar (approximately 4 grams) per 8 ounces of water, which aligns with the World Health Organization's (WHO) recommended oral rehydration solution (ORS) formula."[11] Notice how high that recommendation is on salt.

Now, let's talk about balancing these two. The FDA and the American Heart Association recommend consuming only 2.3 grams of salt per day.[12] Yet, the FDA recommends

---

that people consume 50 grams of added sugar a day. If you follow the math, the World Health Organization's recommendation for hydration is much heavier on salt. Yet in the US, salt is villainized in our diet recommendations, and the allowed sugars are much higher. It's very strange indeed.

Next, let's get into my research for this book. Every book I read on longevity, fasting, nutrition, or autoimmune diseases stated that we need to eat less refined sugars. Every. Single. One. Coincidence? I think not. Yet, only one book discussed salt. Enter one of the four books, and arguably the most important, that I read on my research journey. In his book entitled *The Salt Fix*,[13] Dr. James DiNicolantonio boldly states that, for most of us, more salt is better than less, and plainly, sugar is worse. He covers how we are told to eat less and move more. That strategy does NOT work for most people! He also states that sugar causes most of the chronic diseases we currently have today, not salt. And yet, many US dietary guidelines have always pushed sugars and villainized salt. Let's just say that, in general, I agree with Dr. DiNicolantonio on this as well.

The doctor also includes more information about what salt helps heal, which was instrumental for me with one of these issues. He argues that there is no sound scientific evidence to support the correlation between salt and high blood pressure. His book recommends a low-carb, high-salt diet for most people to manage their weight. Low salt levels can also cause symptoms of cold hands and feet and lightheadedness when standing after sitting for long periods of time. He goes on to talk about how without salt, we can't live, the risk of death is higher with low salt intake rather than high, and that low salt levels are the cause for low sex drive! Crazy. I think you get the point: Salt should not be villainized like it is. But the one solution that had the most impact for me was that salt helps heal reoccurring staph infections.

Staph is short for *Staphylococcus*, a type of bacteria that can cause potentially serious and recurring infections once it's introduced to the bloodstream. Staph is commonly found on the skin and in the nose. About 10 years ago, during one of my sessions on my first sleeve tattoo, I contracted a staph infection so bad I had to be hospitalized and have emergency surgery on my elbow. Subsequently, for years, I had to take antibiotics about every six months to keep the infections from recurring. My specialist told me that these reoccurrences would be lifelong. The skin on my face also became seriously prone to fungal acne on my forehead; the staph also increased the appearance of wrinkles because of this. Needless to say, it was brutal.

Over a year ago, I began to incorporate some of the doctor's advice, just not at the same scale. For sugar, he recommends limiting total added sugar to no more than 30 grams per day—less than the FDA's 50-gram recommendation. Ideally, no more than 20 grams of your daily sugar intake should come from added sugars. He also advises cutting out ALL sugary drinks (since liquid sugar is the worst) and avoiding artificial sweeteners completely. On all non-cheat days, I agree with him and typically follow this advice on sugar. When it comes to salt, he claims that we should be eating 2 to 3 teaspoons of salt a day. For reference: 1 teaspoon of salt = 5.69 grams, 2 = 11.38 grams, and 3 = 17.07 grams. Personally, I think the top end of that recommendation is madness, at nearly 7.5 times the current FDA daily recommended value. I simply disagree with him here. Too much salt can still cause real issues like headaches, heart palpitations from disrupting the sodium and calcium balance, bloating and digestive problems, sleep disturbances, and even long-term heart complications, among others. I seriously recommend not following this advice.

It's all about balance here. I personally recommend starting small with the salt, only increasing your intake by 1/8 teaspoon or .5 grams a day, as well as increasing your water intake slightly (say 4 ounces) each day until optimizing what works best for you. I'll further discuss the salt types in the chapter summary. Once you begin seeing a visible improvement in your skin's elasticity and hydration, along with feeling like you're not having any issues caused by the salt, you should be good on non-exercise days. If you're exercising or losing lots of sweat for whatever reason, ensure you follow the WHO's oral rehydration recommendation in general.

Since doing this, my skin looks more youthful and hydrated, and I have not had a recurrence of a staph infection since. Incredible! Who knew the solution to one of my most pestering and persistent health problems was sitting on my countertop the entire time? It's also a huge benefit to have my skin looking more youthful, less acne-prone, and simply healthier! True hydration optimization for the win.

IN SUMMARY:

- Experiment with incorporating less sugars (target: 30 grams per day) and more salts (target: .5-1 grams per day) into your regular diet. Approximately increase your water intake by at least 4 ounces per .5 grams of salt.

- For the types of sugars, limit yourself to only 20 grams of added sugars a day. For the types of salt, begin with either coarse kosher salt or sea salt, whichever you respond to best. You can also incorporate iodized salt every three days or so if you follow a diet without much dairy or seafood and you're exhibiting some signs of an iodine deficiency.

- A personal recommendation would be to take the .5-1 gram of salt about an hour after your last meal of the day with a glass of water. This ensures the last thing you consume is hydrating. You can even try adding the salt underneath your tongue when you consume it for increased efficacy. Or, feel free to simply add additional salts to foods you don't enjoy eating, like steamed veggies. Adjust as necessary based on your results.

Even when I started my writing journey, I never would've imagined I would write such an in-depth chapter on sugar and salt. The next chapter, however, I could totally see myself writing about. Let's get into a topic hardly any of the other books I read wanted to discuss: drugs and alcohol. No real Margaritaville would be complete without it, amirite? Let’s waste away in the next chapter.

Chapter Six: Margaritaville Part 2 – Alcohol and Substances

Yes, alcohol and substances. I can just feel the controversy that may brew from writing this chapter. Everyone has strong opinions and advice regarding this topic. There's lots of contradictory info out there about them, too. Most books hardly touch on this topic. If they do, it's typically for therapeutic or addiction reasons. We will discuss one different drug in particular in the next chapter—that substance is an illegal one, though. I will only be addressing the two main legal ones in this chapter, as they are all I do or have done in the past. I believe it will still incite emotions and opinions around it either way. Since I have rather unique experiences with them, I decided to write about them here. You may not agree with some of my positions, but my hope is that you're open to thinking about why you have yours. Here we go.

As you probably guessed, the two substances I'll primarily be writing about are alcohol and marijuana. I have my opinions on hard or illegal drugs, too, but I'll save them until later. Several studies out now blame alcohol as the third leading cause of preventable cancer cases. There are also brain doctors who swear that even mild alcohol use causes several issues. There is also varying research on marijuana that says it negatively impacts sleep and brain function as well. It's ironic. Before, there were studies that showed that one glass of wine a day was good for you. I personally think there's no way a study can fully attribute these factors solely to substances alone, as there are so many other factors in play.

There are many reasons people are susceptible to cancer, struggle with sleep, and experience accelerated brain aging. The largest one, in my opinion, is diet. What about the outliers in these studies? People who drink every single day and live to be in their 90s and 100s? But let's just assume for a moment that these studies are 100% true. Are you going to stop, or have you tried to stop because of them? My guess for most is a resounding no.

I personally have a rather rare and amazing story with alcohol. After my aforementioned kidney donation surgery, I had major complications and developed stage 3 chronic kidney disease. Given the rarity of the situation, the National Kidney Foundation wanted additional data on my case. I began seeing a high-level, specialized nephrologist and worked with him to see if we could improve my situation. I was initially prescribed a common blood pressure medication, but I experienced side effects and saw no improvement in my kidney function numbers.

Then, the doctor decided to give me a different and rather unique prescription. He replaced the meds with…beer. He told me to increase my water intake throughout the day and then drink three to four beers an evening as a natural diuretic. In simpler terms, it was to assist in opening up the blood vessels of my remaining kidney and help me pee more. Crazy, right? I didn't drink much beer or any alcohol back then, frankly, only a few nights a month with friends. But I had a rather healthy relationship with it, so I thought, "What the heck?" What's crazier than this prescription is that…it actually worked! Immediately and steadily, my kidney numbers showed continual improvement, all the way until I returned to normal range numbers. I felt back to normal, too. All of this occurred in just over a year. It also helped me with my social introversion. Here are a few words I never thought any human would ever write: Beer saved my remaining kidney.

Some years later, after some life challenges set in, beer became…not so productive. I began drinking more than this recommendation during relationship challenges and work issues. Needless to say, it did not help. I never ran into formal alcohol-related issues with the law, but I got extremely close. It was a wake-up call. So, I took breaks from drinking—months off at a time. After getting through the tough times, I was able to resume drinking responsibly to where I am today. I drink three to four beers a few days a week and then stay sober the rest of the time. Once a month or on a special occasion, I'll get into a few more than that, but you see the point: moderation.

Now, on to weed. Mary Jane. The ganja. I've never been an everyday or wake-and-bake guy—more of an every-other-day-or-so guy, mostly in the afternoon and evenings. I only started doing it after it became legal in my state and just for fun. It was always edibles; I rarely ever smoked. I definitely found it beneficial in calming my overthinking. But much like alcohol, I ran into my issues with it. Namely, it really hampered my productivity. Some people can do it and work their faces off—but not me. It also caused me to be rather emotional and sensitive to things when I was coming off of it. After years of being a rather regular user, I'm not using it at all these days. I just have too much to get done. In contradiction to the research, though, I never really had any of the issues they claim, including trouble sleeping when I used it.

I wanted to provide context here for my forthcoming recommendations. And as a disclaimer, I also think it's tough to tell people what to do with substances, especially if they have a history of family abuse. At the end of the day, I think people should and will just do what's best for them, including you. I have several friends who enjoy them and several friends who are sober. I love them just the same. It's how it should be. Just know that if you ponder these things, you're not alone. These are complicated subjects; just be sure you never end up pressured into anything you don't want to do.

IN SUMMARY:

- Everything in moderation: Too much of anything is bad, and developing self-control to enjoy them is just fine as long as you don't have a greater medical issue or addiction problems that forces you to abstain altogether.

- Always lean toward drinking alcohol with food. Several studies show it's much safer that way for various reasons.

- Look at yourself honestly and determine if a substance is serving you and your goals. If it's not, make a change. If making a change is hard, get some help. And fuck people who shame people for getting help.

- Generally, the best advice is to avoid substances if you're going through a tough season in life. They're much more beneficial and enjoyable during times of contentment.

That felt like a really heavy chapter. But, in my opinion, it had to be written. Addressing complicated issues is kind of turning into my thing now. As you'll see in some of the upcoming chapters, I'm planning to get way more controversial than this on some recommendations. Even I am not immune to getting excited at the thought. Let's keep going!

Chapter Seven: Autoimmunity

"Health is not valued till sickness comes." – Thomas Fuller[14]

Ahh, here's another semi-corny quote to start off a chapter. I absolutely love loathing that about books. But as an official member of the Author Club, I feel somewhat compelled to conform occasionally. This is a wise one, though. Supposedly, this dude lived in the 1600s and was a 'clergyman.' You get five points if you knew what that is without looking it up. I wonder if he had autoimmune issues, too? It's estimated that autoimmune disorders affect approximately 1 in 10 people (out of those who report it). I have suffered from my fair share, too, so I choose to write about it. I am also fascinated by it. Many of the previous chapters add up to my thoughts on this one. The main issue I have seen and agree with another book on the topic is that healthcare providers typically disregard root causes in favor of symptom management. Let's dive into why that's problematic.

In the book *The Autoimmune Cure* written by Sara Szal Gottfried, MD, she shares several tidbits of wisdom and recommendations from her area of expertise.[15] She warns that you should not take pharmaceuticals for autoimmune issues, as only 1 in 3 people benefit from it. Her take is that autoimmune issues are a perfect storm of stress and aging. Furthermore, trauma is the cause of this disease. She goes on to claim that trauma and hormones are the root cause of these issues and leaky gut syndrome. Since the intestinal mucus layer refreshes every two to five days, diet is the biggest cause. To deal with all of this, she recommends both elimination diets and therapy, along with psychedelic drugs to "cure" this disease. As you can probably guess, I agree with some of this, and I have a real problem with the other.

First off, even though I don't believe it's included in her book, I personally think this only applies to non-physiological cases of autoimmune disease. This would not include cases like MS (multiple sclerosis), where the protective myelin sheath covering the nerve fibers within the cord becomes damaged. I fully believe that once a major physical change in the body like that occurs, medical and pharmaceutical intervention is required. I am simply not certain enough to determine if that can be restored by my process, nor do I think it's safe to try. I am not a doctor, but eventually, I would like to chat with one about these instances, as my grandma had, and a few of my close friends have, MS. Now, I will get into what I believe happened in my instance of autoimmune disease.

My story started when trying to pinpoint what my diagnosis was. My physician was unable to pinpoint it between lupus, rheumatoid arthritis, Crohn's, or Hashimoto's disease, as I had symptoms from all of them. Here's a list of the most prevalent symptoms I was experiencing:

- Periodic butterfly rash on my checks and intermittent watery stools
- Low blood cell counts and severe night sweats when sleeping
- Dry skin, dry eyes, and thinning hair
- Fatigue, muscle cramps, anemia, and weight loss
- Sensitivity to cold, headaches, and minor memory problems
- Various patches of psoriasis and the skin on all my fingertips randomly peeling off to the point of bleeding

As you can see, I was a full-blown hot mess express two years ago. That last one really pissed me off because it kept me from playing golf with the homies a couple of times. I was also super stressed out at the time; I had just broken up with my live-in girlfriend and concurrently started a new job in the same month. My symptoms continued for months after as well. The good ol' clergyman was right—I needed to address what was going on.

In lieu of continuing to depend on my PCP to figure all of this out, I once again went back to my health clinic and worked with my personalized health coach, Dom, to straighten this out. Going back to *The Autoimmune Cure* and her recommendation of elimination diets, something struck me. I decided to have Dom run another full micronutrient panel and found several more nutrients in which I was newly deficient. Instead of limiting foods, I decided to target directly where my deficiencies were. The result was nothing short of amazing. So now, let's get into *why*.

One day, while driving my 21-year-old daughter to college (CU has limited parking), I mentioned this chapter to her. She's quite the brilliant kiddo, a pre-med student majoring in psychology. She knows my story well and told me to look into epigenetics. If you don't know what that is, you're not alone. I didn't either. It turns out that epigenetics refers to how your behaviors and environment can cause changes that affect the way your genes work. Unlike genetic changes (mutations), epigenetic changes are reversible and do not change the sequence of DNA bases, but they can change how your body reads a DNA sequence.[16] There are four main epigenetic mechanisms, including DNA methylation (there's that word again), histone modification, chromatin remodeling, and noncoding RNA (ncRNA), which exert different effects on metabolic diseases. [17]

With all of that said, here's my more simplified life-hacker theory on what the fuck I experienced and think happens with stress-induced autoimmune diseases.

1. Stress depletes micronutrients quickly, both (fat) stored and water-soluble.

2. Micronutrient-depleted cells change how your body reads a DNA sequence.

3. To reverse the changes, restore the micronutrients, both in the cells and water-soluble, to restore the body's ability to optimally read the DNA sequence.

That's my oversimplified hypothesis. I'm also basing that shit on some science, as you can see. I also believe that since I had the MTHFR gene mutation, the symptoms were more difficult to pin down. With that said, what I know is that with the exception of some very minor and small psoriasis spots (which I am now close to solving during the book's editing phase), I have resolved every single symptom on that list without the use of drugs or pharmaceuticals. Amazing. Let's get into the chapter summary and the hypothesized solution.

IN SUMMARY:

- Your body has the amazing ability to heal itself when it's given the proper nutrients. I believe that most environment-modified or trauma-caused autoimmune issues can be dealt with by a micronutrient intake analysis discussed in the diet chapter, then subsequent corresponding diet modifications and stress management.

- Extract yourself from stressful situations as much as possible and ensure that during unavoidable ones, you make it a point to keep your nutrient levels up where you are susceptible to depletion. Also, think about temporarily increasing exercise during stressful times to convert any nervous energy.

- Again, I'll reiterate that you should rotate different foods regularly in your diet and avoid eating the same types of foods all the time. Mix in various meatless and vegan days occasionally and 24- to 48-hour fasts a few times a year. All of this helps to reset and keep the gut's mucus layer healthy.

- Fuck doing hard drugs like psychedelics to solve autoimmune issues. Try my way first and see what happens. My guess is that you'll be amazed by the results. Marijuana was also beneficial for a time period to help calm my anxiety and lessen the severity of the symptoms around this, too, but this is certainly not required.

Enter Mr. Mackey via Southpark fame to say, "Drugs are bad, *m'kay*." I kid. In all seriousness, this is an issue that is close to my heart, and if it's close to yours, too, I hope you appreciate my take. Autoimmune diseases are awful, and anything we can do to prevent them all-naturally is nothing short of awesome.

Up next is another emotional chapter for me. I promise this book will continue to get even better as we go. And I can't wait to keep writing it for you! Thanks for coming along on this journey; it means the world to me. Next up: doctors and pharmaceuticals.

Chapter Eight: Getting Real About Doctors and Pharmaceuticals

One might assume that since my mother's ultimate demise came at the hands of the direction of doctors and by way of pharmaceuticals that I am getting ready to begin a bashing session. Far from it—I realize how many lives are saved by doctors and pharmaceutical drugs. I look up to quite a few doctors and respect the hell out of what they do. As evidenced by this book, I take from their research and recommendations all the time. But, thank God I am not one. So much of what I love to do as part of my ventures is to implement various experts' research simultaneously to bring you the ultimate outcomes that are otherwise not achievable. However, your outcomes of these relationships with both doctors and pharma will undoubtedly be one of the highest contributors to satisfaction in your health and life. There are lessons to be learned in my mom's story. Being cautious of what you put into your body is massive, and so is a change in philosophy with healing the body.

In my research, my personal favorite book was that of a 102-year-old doctor. You see, I have a deep appreciation for old-school things and advice from old souls. The wisdom in their words is palpable. Enter *A Well Lived Life* by the centenarian mother of holistic medicine herself, Dr. Gladys McGarey.[18] Of the four books I quote in this book, this one is

---

the best. I highly recommend you give it a read. Here are her six actionable secrets to enjoying lives that are long, happy, and purpose-driven:

1. Spend your energy wildly.
2. All life needs to move.
3. You are here for a reason.
4. You are never alone.
5. Everything is your teacher.
6. Love is the most powerful medicine.

They're all profound, to say the least. Some of my favorite sentiments from the book were as follows:

- Nobody goes through life without experiencing how hard it can be.
- We have a choice in life: Will we direct our attention toward love or fear?
- Pain is the best teacher: Even if we can't make something easy, is there anything we can do to make it easier?
- We can start (to tackle problems) by resisting the urge to fight.

- Look for false beliefs you may have about avoiding risks or not having enough, and look for the lessons available to us when we feel broken.

- Ask what you put in before looking to get anything out.

There are many more, but the establishment of this philosophy is what's truly important here. It's what I believe so much is lost in our present-day mentality to healing. It's just that—our mentality. Our mindset. In lieu of some struggling, we want a quick fix. Her advice discusses that it's okay to struggle sometimes. And that struggle can be the true blessing. Envisioning a way forward where we can ask ourselves, 'What can I change?' instead of 'What medicine will fix this?' is what I took away as one of the main points from the book. Before reading it, it was a philosophy I wholeheartedly believed in. She explains it beautifully and in a way that helps you understand why.

Getting back to traditional doctors, they can be very useful and downright imperative in the right context, as can pharma. Your PCP can help finish the painting of your health that is started by the health clinics and diagnose the need for major surgeries. As we all know, sometimes physiological changes occur in our bodies and can only be corrected with invasive surgery. Drugs are a necessity in many instances as well and don't regularly cause issues whatsoever. For example, look at anesthesia, antibiotics, and synthetic insulin, just to name a few.

Then, there's holistic medicine. It can help us address many problems as well. In my humble opinion, they should overwhelmingly be preferred as the starting point for most common ailments. Like cranberry juice for a UTI, oregano oil capsules to fight a cold virus, or thyme leaves for a yeast infection or build up in infected mucus, they very much have their uses until you can determine the root cause of the reoccurrence. Learning to balance these approaches can have a profound impact on your approach to healing the body as well. Also, keep that in mind the next time you reach for the medicine shelf at your local grocery store or pharmacy.

IN SUMMARY:

- Own your general health first by trying to solve symptoms via diet and exercise before turning to PCP pharmaceuticals.

- Use PCPs for less expensive routine labs in problematic areas once they have been targeted by a health clinic. Provide them with the health clinic data to show them your starting points, and watch them become happy to assist.

- As a general rule, avoid unnecessary pharmaceuticals as much as possible. Only interface with them as needed, like when there's a diagnosed physiological reason for doing so.

- There are good and safe pharmaceutical drugs out there. Always know the risks and side effects people experience with drugs before taking one. Try to always stick to drugs that have been on the market for long periods of time and have a strong history of very low side effects.

- Always check for and implement holistic alternatives for minor or temporary health issues over pharma solutions first.

Once you begin implementing these practices in dealing with your health issues, a sense of satisfaction sets in. Learning to appreciate doctors and pharmaceuticals for what's really important (surgeries, physiological ailments, etc.) is the key to appreciating them again if you have developed a difficult relationship with them. Everything plays its part. Knowing what's best suited for each role can make all the difference.

Now, let's get into the chapters where *I* am the expert. I've been waiting patiently for this. My guess is that if you chose to read the entire book from start to finish instead of jumping to these chapters like I'm sure many will, I commend your patience, too! As important as the first half of this book is, it wouldn't be complete without what's to come. It's with no further ado, I say to you: Let's fucking go!

Chapter Nine: Face Facts – The Science of Physical Attraction

Much like the diet versus exercise conversation, I have a clear preferred position in 'looks maxing' too. Many people spend their efforts in the gym, trying to craft the perfect *body* they think will make them look the best in order to attract their desired partner. There's one problem, though: science. Specifically, the science of physical attraction. While someone's body and level of fitness is a factor and we've already covered how I like to address it initially (slimming with diet), I can attest from personal experience where the results lie. There's plenty of great info on how to build muscle and even how to introduce exogenous hormone utilization for bulking, etc., on YouTube. That is not my area of expertise, nor do I practice it. Let's cover why you should face the facts of science and start honing that beautiful dome piece of yours, shall we?

After the science, I will speak a bit about my personal experience. While it's difficult to put an exact percentage on it, research suggests that facial attractiveness plays a significant role in overall physical attraction, possibly even outweighing body attractiveness in some cases. In essence:[19]

- **Faces are a major factor in attraction.** Studies have shown that facial cues are often given more weight than body cues when judging overall attractiveness.

- **Facial features influence perceptions.** Features like facial symmetry, youthfulness, and averageness (approaching the average facial configuration of a population) are often considered attractive across cultures.
- **Individual preferences matter.** While some aspects of facial attractiveness might be universal, individual preferences and experiences also play a significant role in who we find attractive.

Since we have already covered improving youthfulness with skin hydration by improving your diet and increasing your salt intake in previous chapters, we will dig deeper into facial symmetry and averageness.

- **Facial Symmetry:** Facial symmetry has been found to increase ratings of attractiveness in human faces. More symmetrical faces are perceived as more attractive in both males and females, although facial symmetry plays a larger role in judgments of attractiveness concerning female faces. Studies have shown that nearly symmetrical faces are considered highly attractive compared to asymmetrical ones. [20]

- **Facial Averageness:** In physical attractiveness studies, averageness describes the physical beauty that results from averaging the facial features of people of the same gender and approximately the same age. The majority of averageness studies have focused on photographic overlay studies of human faces, in which images are morphed together. The term "average" is used strictly to denote the technical definition of the mathematical mean. An averaged face is not unremarkable but is, in fact, quite good-looking. Nor is it typical in the sense of being common or frequently occurring in the population—though it appears familiar, it is typical in that it serves as a strong example of a face representative of the overall category. A possible evolutionary explanation for averageness is koinophilia, in which sexually reproducing animals seek mates with primarily average features because extreme and uncommon features are likely to indicate disadvantageous mutations. [21]

  A University of Toronto study found that the facial proportions of celebrities like Jessica Alba were close to the average of all female profiles.

Now, you might be asking yourself, "Why is all of this important?" The answer is simple. If you really want to improve your looks, *this* is how you do it: Improve your face.

While a certain degree of your facial features pertaining to averageness are genetic and static, you can still improve the appearance of most of them. For example, interocular distance is the measurement between your two pupils, and not much can be changed there. However, there are approximately 43 muscles in the face and 20 muscles in the neck. These muscles can be honed to alter your facial appearance, namely in the nose, jaw, eye shape and mouth areas. There are also certain bones you can move to contribute to this effort as well, which is a widely accepted concept in medical science. The amount of beneficial change you can create in these measurements and improved symmetry in these areas is nothing short of amazing.

In my time being single since my divorce in 2015, I have done my fair share of dating, albeit as a heterosexual male. Without dragging you through all the details, I went from being unable to get but a few dates a year when I started to now not being able to handle all of the messages I receive from women anytime I join an online dating app. I am probably one of the few men in the world who has ever experienced this varying level of polarity. The cool thing about this is that I know exactly how I did it. And in the next few chapters, I am going to write about it to help you!

IN SUMMARY:

- Facial attractiveness has as much, if not more, of a profound impact on attracting a romantic partner than body attractiveness.
- The factors of facial features like symmetry, youthfulness, and averageness are often considered attractive across cultures.
- You can improve the appearance of these factors by enhancing your nutrition, repositioning certain bones and working certain muscles in the face and neck.

Get ready because you are about to read one of the wildest stories you'll ever hear, and it contains the keys to improving your facial attractiveness!

Chapter Ten: Story of a Sloped-Chined, Crooked Jaw

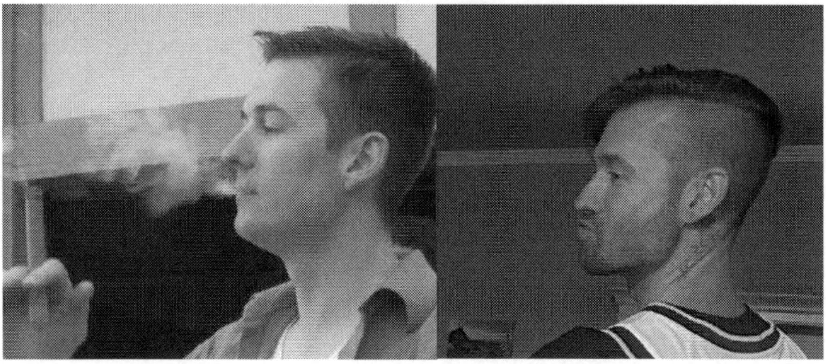

The first picture on the left is me, approximately 12 years ago. The picture on the right is me about a year ago. If you're listening to the audiobook version, please pause the book and quickly head over to @thoroughwayne on Instagram, and I'll have the picture pinned there. You can clearly see just how different I look, and I'm routinely told I don't even look like the same person now. This journey and seeing people asking for help on TikTok videos and in comments of jaw videos is the greatest motivation for me in writing this book. Per Google, I currently know more than doctors and specialists in this area. Remarkably, I achieved this result without any surgery whatsoever. Back in the day, I wanted to at least try to accomplish what so many say is impossible…and then I did. I was able to turn my greatest weakness into my greatest strength, and it changed my entire life. I am assuming that at least a few of you will be able to relate to exactly what happened in the early part of my journey and my awful diagnosis.

In my mid-20s, I started getting horrible migraine headaches, astigmatism in only my right eye, and a clicking in my jaw when I opened it. By the time I was 30 years old, I could hardly open my mouth, and as you can see, I had a full-on sloped chin with no profile or jawline to speak of. In 2016, my opening got so bad that I finally decided to see a jaw specialist/orthodontist. He measured my bite opening at a startling 12 millimeters, slightly larger than half an inch. Even he couldn't believe it at the time. Needless to say, it was awful in so many ways. Note: I was told by my orthodontist that the average opening for an adult is 30 to 35mm, but a quick Google search shows it's actually 40 to 60mm, which seems more accurate to me. That context is startling to me looking back.

He then referred me to an oral surgeon who ordered tons of fancy X-rays of my head, jaw, and face. Afterward, this is what I was diagnosed with: hemifacial microsomia. My first thought was probably similar to one you'd have, 'What the fuck is that?' Here's the formalized medical description:

- Hemifacial microsomia is a common congenital facial difference that causes asymmetric development of the face. Hemifacial has been called many terms, such as Goldenhar syndrome and oculo-auriculo-vertebral spectrum. They are all the same condition. This condition may affect all structures of the face but most commonly causes asymmetry of the eyes, jaws, ears, muscles, and

> nerves that allow a patient to smile and the soft tissues of the face. [22]

I've also seen this referred to online as 'facial or cranial torsion.' The research I've conducted shows that they're effectively relative conditions that cause facial and cranial asymmetry but have different fundamental causes. In my case, the condition was largely caused by one side of my face and jawbone (right side) growing several millimeters longer than the other. At birth, I was also pulled out of my mom in a way that caused a massive bump on my head, and I suspect this was also a somewhat relative cause. A doctor I spoke with at a golf course years ago confirmed this as a probable contributing factor as well. These issues caused the center of my chin to sit severely asymmetrical to the center of my face, also creating imbalances in my nose and up to my ears. A funny note: Upon diagnosis the oral surgeon told me that 98% of people diagnosed with this condition were middle-aged African American women and that I was in the "lucky" 2% of all other cases. Lucky me!

Clearly, I had a major problem on my hands. When we discussed treatment options, he told me that if I were his brother or a close family member, he would tell me not to do surgery. Generally speaking, I am also anti-cosmetic surgery or just surgery in general unless there are extreme outlier cases or conditions to justify it. One would certainly classify this as extreme, but I also sided against surgery. His formal advice was to get braces to slightly improve the opening and just deal with it, as there was no other cure or way to improve it. So, at first, that's what I did. Throughout 2017 and 2018, I wore braces as an adult for nearly two years. It did help some—moving my opening from 12mm to 21mm (a little over one inch) and slightly reducing the slope of my chin—but not by much. When googling how facial asymmetry is treated, this is what I found:

- **Braces**: Braces can be used to fix facial asymmetry.
- **Surgery**: Surgery may be needed for more serious cases of facial asymmetry.
- **Plastic Surgery**: Plastic surgery or jaw surgery may be needed for uneven muscles or bone structure issues. [23]

As evidenced by my bone structure issues, I was, and still probably am, medically in the severest of categories. Enter early 2021: I had gone through my last retainer/nightguard (I'm a grinder), so I went back to the orthodontist to be fitted for a new one. The young woman fitting it asked, "Have you been doing your jaw exercises for your TMJ?" I responded no because I hadn't really been having any pain. Braces did help with that. So, on my way out, she gave me a sheet with two exercises, basically showing how to stretch the mandible. Don't worry—that's not my big advice, and I still don't use these exercises to this day.

The idea of exercises did pique my interest, though. It opened my mind to change in that way, and for that, I am forever grateful. At first, I tried a few different exercises I made up myself. One of the first ones I tried was sticking my bottom jaw out 20 or 30 times a day; all that ended up doing was causing the bottom hinge on the right side of my jaw to get sore over and over with no improvement. So, I scrapped it. I took a few weeks off, and then came seemingly the most obvious and simultaneously dumb idea I ever had.

I thought to myself, *I want to open my jaw wider, right? What if I just tried to open it over and over, every single day?* It seemed counterintuitive…I couldn't do it, right? Why continue to try? But, instead of believing that judgment and letting that thought sit, I made the deal with myself I spoke about in Chapter 2. Every single day for at least a month, I was going to try. Ironically, the protocol I set for myself is the one I still largely follow to this day. As soon as I woke up, I would hit the bathroom, make my bed, and then try to open my mouth as wide as I could for 100 reps. After day one, nothing. Day two, same thing. One-week, same story. I still just tried and tried, every single day. Two weeks, nada. But one month? I noticed an ever-so-*slight* change. And it wasn't in my jaw opening…I'll explain.

One summer weeknight, a month after starting the opening exercises, I was hanging out with my 14-year-old son and his best friend T, watching some Nuggets basketball. I was drinking a few beers, and the kids thought it'd be fun to throw on some rap music instead of listening to the commentators. Then, one of my favorite all-time songs came on, Tupac's "Me Against the World." I thought this simple moment deserved to be captured by a selfie video for my Instagram story, seeing as how my son and I were somehow enjoying the same music for the first time! In the video, I noticed that my eyes looked more connected than they had in years. There was a slight 'twinkle,' if you will, in them again. My right eye had always been more shut compared to my left since these jaw issues started, too, and now my right eye looked slightly more open, more symmetrical.

Oh fuck, I thought. I came to the conclusion that not working these muscles was causing the issues with my vision in my right eye! It felt like a breakthrough. So, I kept going. About two months in, I decided to start informally measuring my opening. Since our refrigerator doesn't have a water filter on it, we largely used to drink bottled water. I started using bottle caps from the different kinds of water bottles as goals to hit. I started at the Arrowhead 16oz bottle cap. Then, after about two and a half months, I was able to get a Smart Water 32oz cap—a 2mm improvement! After that, it just continued. I kept going, experiencing 1 or 2 millimeters of progress every two to three months. After a year of just five minutes of exercises a day, I could fit two fingers, or about 35 millimeters—amazing! Insert your favorite inappropriate fitting-things-into-your-mouth joke here.

After about a year though, I plateaued. I was stuck at 35mm for over a year and a half. This is where the story starts to get pretty wild. After two and a half years of jaw exercises, including adding a few additional ones, I looked like a different person. My face was far more slender, and I had an actual jawline…as evidenced by the after photo above. In the fall of 2023, I was single for nearly a year when I was notified by someone that a reality television show that shall remain nameless was doing some casting in my city. I was encouraged to apply by said someone, so I decided, "What the heck?" and did. After months of casting duties, to my surprise, they offered me a contract to appear on the show in three months. Given I'd be the oldest person to ever appear in the history of this show at 41, I didn't really think this was possible. Needless to say, I was kind of freaking out.

I'll finish the rest of my offshoot TV story in the forthcoming dating rant chapter, but as you can see, I had some additional motivation to try and improve. Enter yet another seemingly unrelated yet totally related side story: A childhood buddy of mine and I have played golf since we were kids. A few years ago, he built a fully transitional golf simulator in his garage. Every time we play on it, I take a few videos of our swing and throw them on my Instagram story just to laugh at ourselves. I promise I don't post a lot (yet), but this is the only time I really see myself externally—so that's how it's related. I noticed that my posture was pretty bad in one of the videos during the three-month period I was waiting for filming. And now, I had the motivation to do something about it. I came to find out that this would relate right back to my jaw and my vision in the strangest of ways.

Many massage therapists always say our bodies are very connected. For example, a muscle could be hurting in one area because of a problem in an entirely different part of your body. My continued story is certainly evidence of that! One evening, while I was doomscrolling Instagram reels, I came across a guy doing posture exercises and decided to throw them into my typical jaw exercise routine, as they only added about a minute. I did them every day for about two months and saw a noticeable improvement in the appearance of my posture. Then, one of the weirdest nights of my life happened.

Late at night, while sitting at my computer, the right side of my jaw was uncharacteristically aching. I went to open my mouth to stretch it, and then…POP! I heard one of the loudest popping noises I had ever heard in my life. The entire right side of my face was numb with pain for a solid minute, and accompanying it was a piercing buzzing noise in my right ear. "Did I blow my eardrum?" I thought. I waited for a few minutes. The pain subsided, and the sound went away. I went to open my jaw again, and this time, there was another pop that hurt but not as bad. I opened it again and measured it. It jumped another 5mm or so! I couldn't believe it. I knew that hinge had been closed for about 15 years. It started to hurt after opening it a few more times, so I decided to rest it for the night. This is where the strangest part of the story happens. Yes, it gets weirder…I know, right?

While I was sleeping, I had an odd dream of being able to see things around my hometown like when I was a kid. When I woke up, I went to the bathroom like usual, and out of the corner of my eye, I caught myself in the mirror. When I looked at myself, I hardly recognized my reflection! My vision had also been modified for several years because of the closed jaw hinge. I remember people telling me that I looked different, but my reflection still looked the same to me. That's because I was only seeing things flat—basically in two dimensions—with little to no depth perception. After this hinge popped back into place, my depth perception finally returned. Needless to say, I had an emotional reaction. Ironically, this morning happened one year ago to the day of writing this.

Now, on to why this happened. Clearly, there was a tendon connected all the way down to my shoulder or possibly further down in my back that had gone too far forward due to my bad posture and needed to be worked back into place to allow my opening to fully return. "But what about the additional length on that right side?" you might be thinking. I have a couple of theories here: Either the muscles and tendons in my face adapted around it to make it work, or the bones in my face slightly widened to account for it on that side. Without additional X-rays, there's no way to know for sure. I will probably never pay for them either, so I'll likely never know.

Regardless, the combination of several varying exercises along with orthodontic treatment largely solved this issue for me. And I think it will be for anyone suffering from similar issues, too. The key is that it's multifaceted. There are multiple interrelated problems that all need to be addressed simultaneously to correct these issues, and that's why nobody has figured it out until now. The next chapter will simply be the general process for you to reference. Feel free to also adapt and modify specifically for your issues. Never be afraid to try an exercise for a while, too; you never know what could help.

I must also comment on the other channels and pages I've seen posting different advice on how to address some of these issues, like people using their hands to work on pulling different parts of their gums, etc. While I think these things *may* be somewhat effective, it seems far too single-minded to me. I truly believe that if you just do exercises to target the functionality of these areas instead, the muscle—and possibly even the bones—will naturally follow. Nearly all of my facial symmetry has returned after years of these exercises, and clearly, I didn't operate on any of my bones. Coincidence? I think not. I believe it's the positioning of the muscles and tendons that largely changes. How else could I have accomplished this?

Fast forward to today, now when I open my jaw after it hasn't been opened for a while, it still pops in that upper right hinge. It slightly moves into place to allow the full opening to take place. Also, when this hinge popped, it had a major impact on my mandible, shifting it down into place. Unfortunately for me, that meant I had to get braces for a third time—the second time as an adult—and I am smack dab in the middle of my treatment while writing these words. What's funny is that when I saw my orthodontist again after 7 years, he did not recognize me at all. I reminded him of this story, and then we measured my bite opening where I started this time before my braces, too…42 mms, which is so cool to me! Hopefully, it'll be even more when I finish treatment. Thankfully, I have always worn my retainer while I have slept for the last seven years, so I only need them for a handful of months this time. But now, when I'm done, I'll finally be fully *done.* I will never stop the exercises, though. I am committed to them for life to avoid this ever happening again!

Thanks for reading my jaw story. I know it's not cool to have these issues, but look what came out of it. I believe God does work in mysterious ways. I am the proof. And now, I want to help you try to achieve your goals. My guess is that the real you is right around the corner, too!

Chapter Eleven: Through the Cracks, Facial Looks Maxing Process

To drastically improve your facial asymmetry/facial torsion and/or jawline as an adult *without major surgery*, you need to do the following exercises in order, which should take no longer than five to six minutes daily while standing with your feet shoulder-width apart. Incorporate other treatments and strategies as recommended. I may link a video with the posture exercises on my TikTok @thoroughwayne if there's enough interest.

1) Posture Exercises

    - Shrug shoulders 10 times, and get loose.
    - Move your head directly back 10 times, creating a double chin each time, and hold the last rep in place for 15 seconds. This exercise is to help decompress the spine.
    - Start with your palms facing behind you. Then, rotate both your hands so that your thumbs point directly behind you, opening your chest for 10 reps.
    - Raise both arms to shoulder level with your forearms and hands pointed straight at the ceiling. Pull your arms back 25 to 35 times.

- Raise both arms to shoulder level and fully extend them with your thumbs pointing back. Make large backward circles (about 1.5 to 2 feet in diameter) with your arms, rotating 25 to 35 times.

2) Jaw Exercises (Note: Rest your tongue during all exercises.)

   - Open your mouth and jaw as wide as you can 25 times, and hold the last rep for 5 seconds.

   - Open your jaw while keeping your mouth narrow and relaxed quickly for 50 reps, emphasizing the muscle underneath your chin at the top of your neck. You should feel some pulling down on your nose too.

   - Open your mouth and jaw as wide as you can again 25 times, and hold the last rep for 30 to 45 seconds.

   - Open your mouth and jaw while sucking in your top and bottom lips while raising your cheeks like you are smiling for 25 to 35 reps, and hold the last rep in place for 15 to 30 seconds.

3) Orthodontic Treatment (Braces) for Asymmetry

- I recommend doing the above exercises concurrently for at least three months to ensure your opening is as wide as possible to avoid having to get braces multiple times. Depending on the severity of your situation (like mine), it may be unavoidable.

- Moving your teeth forward is usually required for accentuating your chin and jawline. When you close your bite, only your back teeth should be making contact in your mouth. It's best to consult your dentist if they think orthodontic treatment is best suited for you or if you can forego it.

- I have also discussed the 'thumb pulling' phenomenon with my orthodontist's staff, and they claim the only benefit to it is the stretching aspect of it. You can search the techniques online and incorporate them as you see fit, but I believe the benefits to be nominal for adults.

4) Addressing Mouth Breathing and Tongue Posture

- Mouth-Taping: There are many videos online about mouth taping to improve your jaw position as you sleep. Many also claim mouth-taping will improve your jawline, but in my opinion and like so many things you see online, this is largely horseshit. But mouth breathing should be addressed to optimize jaw positioning while you sleep and ensure you breathe correctly through your nose.

- You can choose to tape your mouth shut while you sleep, but if you're anything like me, that idea horrifies the shit out of you. I've invented the following hack instead.

- Ensure your neck and back are straight and parallel, and sleep on your side. Slightly slide a second pillow underneath your head pillow next to your neck and below your chin. Do not slide the second bottom pillow past your chin. This should prop up the bottom of your head pillow, creating a bowl shape around your face and keeping your chin propped up to remain closed if it falls open during sleep.

- Rarely sleep on your back to avoid mouth breathing and snoring. Also, be sure to balance time between both sides, as always sleeping on one side can further exacerbate asymmetry. In general, side sleeping supports nose breathing, ensuring proper jaw posture.

- When you are sleeping or not speaking or eating focus on resting the tip of your tongue at the small indention where the top of your mouth starts to turn down (right below your nose). Formalized tongue therapy is now available in various areas now too, but in my research the main point is to literally develop this habit of resting posture where the tongue largely sits on the top of your mouth.

5) Lymph Node Drainage and Weight Loss for Enhancement

- If you are completing Steps 1 to 4 and still aren't pleased by the aesthetic of your jawline, focus on these areas to accentuate it.

- Your lymph nodes can swell outside of a cold for a myriad of reasons, including in certain autoimmune conditions. It's best to target your diet first to ensure you are consuming enough vitamin C (preferably via a low fructose option like lemon water) and are not dealing with excess calcium in your system, etc. Then, work with your health clinic and doctor to determine the root cause if it continues.

- If you are concerned about weight loss, follow the weight management tips in the previous chapters. Hopefully, you have already read them and know what to do!

- You can also incorporate lymph node massages that are featured on several social media platforms, but I do not personally incorporate most of these and am not privy to their effectiveness. I personally only pinch my ears down from top to bottom, pull them back and pull them out from the earlobes for about 20 seconds each or a minute total a day to engage drainage. I find this works well for me and is all I currently practice.

Some overall quick do's and don'ts:

- **Do** make this easy to complete every single day. **Do not** establish a ton of additional time-consuming measures in your process. If you add additional exercises, only add one at a time to determine their effectiveness. Reward yourself or don't allow yourself to do something you enjoy until you complete them every day.

- **Do** push through some pain, discomfort, and cracking noises. Expect some, especially in the beginning. Do not push through major pain, and listen to your body if you need a break for a day.

Pain reduces gradually and will disappear as you continue the exercises. Our bodies, especially our jaws, were intended to move this way!

- **Do not** use additional devices to 'strengthen' your jaw. Most all people do not want to bulk up their face. Slimming accentuates your natural bone structure, which is the optimal formula for improving your face's appearance.

- **Do** take a selfie once a month or so to track progress and check for slight improvements for motivation. Self-esteem improves with results; results come from the consistent daily work. Make the work quick and easy every day, and watch the results come in. All other standard exercise should be partnered with fun things you like to do or a rewarding activity like a hike to see a neat view, etc.

There you have it: the primary way forward to help formulate a jawline without major surgery. Ensure you keep this multifaceted approach, as every part of this process is important to achieving the best results. I can't wait to see some of your before-and-after pics! Now go and get it.

Chapter Twelve: My Rant on Dating and More Attraction Science

In early February 2024, I had two weeks until I was contracted to begin filming on the aforementioned reality show that shall continue to remain nameless for legal reasons. Up to this point, I was instructed to act as if I were *engaged to be married.* I had done so loyally throughout the entire process, a total of six months. There was a problem, though. Neither I nor my lawyer/cousin had heard back from them on any of the details, and we were beginning to become concerned. We reached out for an update. Up to this point, they had been extremely responsive, keeping me updated with feedback from the network's executive staff team and all the way through the contract signing. Then…silence. Nothing. Ghosted. That's the way I found out I wasn't doing the show. I had been rejected in dating before, but this crushed me. All that time lost and prep wasted. The worst part is that we still don't know exactly why.

With my dating story now concluded, it's time to really get cooking. Buckle up, buttercup, because right now, I am going to get real. This chapter will unquestionably be the most controversial, and I predict it will be the most talked about. Warning: I cuss a lot in it, too. I must be honest, I never planned on being a single 40-something. I thought my marriage was going to be for life. Family. However, I was wrong. And by the stats now in this country, I am certainly not alone. And because there's such a lack of knowledge around the fundamental science of attraction, I believe I know why more people are single now than ever. Like so many of the angles in this book, it is also multifaceted. It's time for me to put some people and certain corporations in their place.

In 2021, 25% of 40-year-olds in the United States had never been married, which is a record high. This is a significant increase from 2010, when 20% of forty-year-olds were unmarried.[24] As of July 1, 2023, there were approximately 21 million people in the United States between the ages of 40 and 49. [25] By the numbers, that would have been 4.2 million 40-something singles, based on 2010 percentages, and 5.25 million 40-something singles today. That's more than a million additional single people in that age group alone, in only 11 years. And these numbers don't even account for the divorced people, like myself, who also remain single. These numbers also prove how popular and desirable marriage still is to the overall general population.

There are also countless numbers of data-backed scientific studies on how people with marital partners end up living significantly longer lives. The younger generations are also trending in a dangerously similar and even worse direction to the 40-something statistics, with over a third of them predicted to never get married. I know people will discuss the differences in dating between both men and women, as single women live slightly longer than single men. Regardless of this minute difference and the varying mating strategies each sex has, the life expectancy consequences are

---

relative for both, so I will speak in generalities throughout this chapter pertaining to singlehood. This life expectancy data, made up of facts measured upon death, also clearly negates the results of any opinion-based studies I have seen various women touting online that state the two happiest groups of people are married men and single women. When the fuck are people going to realize that opinion based studies aren't scientific facts?

We have an existential crisis on our hands in the US. You might be thinking the science doesn't pertain to you, but that only factors in how you feel right now. As you age, you experience the depletion of the production of various hormones. Being alone is much more difficult to cope with after this natural depletion. I believe this is why we get feelings of loneliness—it's to protect our future selves from that inevitable pain. If your loneliness is not a genuine choice (meaning you are actively abstaining from and are fully capable of attracting a physically desirable partner who would treat you well in a long-term relationship) and you never experience feelings of being lonely, it will slowly kill you as you age. The science is clear. Yet, you see many people on various online platforms talking about how happy they are being single right now and that they will never date again. Unfortunately, most who continue that path will die an unnecessarily early death.

I believe there are several reasons why dating is fucked up right now, and I will touch on what I believe are the strongest factors currently. And, like I do, I will build the foundation from a scientific research perspective and go from there. In the early 2000s, the TLC network aired a special called *The Science of Attraction*.[26] Even back then, while in a committed relationship, the science fascinated me. I haven't been able to find the exact programming, but I recall how it worked. The foundation of romantic connection is physical attraction, and this is where their experiment started. They took ten men and ten women to partner together with the following rules:

1) Before entering the pairing room, every participant was given a number from 1 to 10, in accordance with traditional attractiveness rating standards.

2) Each participant was told to hold the number on their forehead, and they were not allowed to directly see their number.

3) Then, each participant was told to go into the room and partner with the highest number they could.

Can you guess what happened? The same thing that happens in real life—the eights, nines, and tens figured out they were exactly that really quickly due to all of the requests they had to partner with them! The rest of the individuals subsequently partnered up as well, and the results were fascinating. No one person partnered with anyone outside of two numbers of their number. This meant that the eights did not partner with anyone higher than a ten or lower than a six, and so on for the rest of the participants. This science is foundational to romantic attraction. The study continued to go on to analyze how status, power, and finances influence romantic connections and make it sufficient for a ten to partner with a four if the four was, for example, rich and/or famous. But, since those situations are largely outliers in the real world of dating and dating apps, we will focus on this foundation.

The incoming statements may piss off a lot of people, but it is what it is. Much of my basis is just facts. I'll preface these comments with the context that I have also studied and have a deep knowledge of nearly every substantial online movement in the dating world, various areas of psychology—including evolutionary, reproductive, and personality—as well as extensive personal experience. I don't take this stuff lightly. And succinctly put, I am fascinated by it. The dating marketplace is difficult, largely because it's one of the main areas in life where we cannot validate ourselves unless it's with external feedback from other potential suitors. We need to self-validate ourselves all the time in life, so we get used to it. But now, lots of single people operate in a world of self-deception. Unless you are experiencing several options of attractive people flying at you left, right, and center, you're not as physically attractive as you might think you are. And based on the science, if you're holding out for a very physically attractive person and are outside of two of that potential partner's number, you are simply setting yourself up for failure and, bluntly, an early death.

Then, we need to briefly touch on other realistic factors outside someone's physical attraction. Before you start to talk about your salary at your high-paying job as making you an outlier, let me remind you that unless you're willing to share that money with your partner, nobody gives a fuck. Couple that with complicating any situation with even more external factors like trying to date when having young children, conflicting morals and values, etc., and you've got one major mess on your hands. All of these factors further negate any physical attraction you may have. The dating marketplace will force you to look at your true value for what it really is…from other people's perspective. That is humbling for most, so they avoid it. Living in delusion is an obvious "L" for everyone involved. And I'm just getting started.

Now, enter dating apps. The era of these apps has led to the most single people in the history of the US for a reason. For starters, they add several distractions for those of us who aren't using them solely for external validation. In addition to creating the façade of numerous options, many of the users lie and deceive constantly, which wastes tons of time. Dating app companies also know the aforementioned fundamental science of physical attraction, and they use it against you. First off, they know your score—your *true* physical attractiveness number—as it's validated externally on their apps. They obviously hide that data from everyone. Then, they use it against you by routinely tempting you with the thought of being with a partner that is, in actuality, several points of physical attraction higher than you. They get everyone trying to punch up to a person two or more points higher in physical attractiveness. Then they use that data to keep you coming back and paying for their shitty product that doesn't help you find a long-term relationship. If you're wondering how I know all of this, I am a former IT engineer/architect, so I know how these scumbag companies formulate their algorithms. I also suspect certain ones even plant good-looking people on them to influence your opinion of their product, but I have no concrete evidence to prove this outside of my own personal experience.

It's really as simple as this—if you find a relationship, they lose a customer. Unless we stop using for-pay dating apps, they will just continue running their scam, taking your money, and leaving you single. I already know what you're thinking: *But how am I supposed to meet someone?* That's a good question. Life is busy, and most of us do not have the social means to meet people we would be ordinarily compatible with outside of these digital connections. With that being said, adaptations must be made. In the future, if you must use apps, I would highly recommend only using free versions like Facebook Dating.

If you are looking to increase your scope, there are also free Facebook groups where they plan gatherings for singles to meet in person in larger cities. There are also meetup apps that can help you connect with new people who have common interests or are simply new to a city and are looking for new friends. If you must use a paid app, the only one I'd even slightly recommend is Match.com, as they mostly do not restrict showing certain users from you and allow you to mostly message anyone, and you can search via zip code on the website version. But seriously, fuck for-pay-swiping-based smartphone apps—they're all trash. Only use them if you are in a smaller market where it's all anyone uses, and do so sparingly. Another fun note: Match Group also owns most of those swipe apps, so also proceed with them at your own discretion.

Let's keep going with this bashing session, shall we? Next up: dating advice. *Ugh*, there's so much of it out there, too. Here's my overly controversial opinion on it:

Most all dating advice, especially direct dating advice like telling you what to do, what to say, or how to act, is fucking garbage!

And, I don't care what a person's qualifications are either, whether they're a doctor, psychologist, lawyer, author, or whatever. Let me explain why. Nearly all of it forces you to be essentially incongruent to your actual feelings—or, simply put, fake—and compels you to follow their strategies to achieve a specific result in lieu of formulating a genuine bond. The worst part about it is that it is quite effective in the short term. However, since it's at its core manipulative and built on a superficial foundation of manufactured feelings instead of authenticity, it will lead you to people without similar value systems and character and, therefore, inevitable long-term failure. This also creates huge messes because of the science of new relationships, which I will soon cover. Basically, this advice just wastes your time—and the time of the people you date—by encouraging you to date people you're not compatible with in the long term. Then, it also adds the hurt and pain from those heartbreaks, further closing us off from other future possibilities. It's tragic for those of us who actually want a meaningful long-term relationship.

What's worse is that specific advice, like approaching random attractive people in public or at the grocery store, truly gets me upset. Like, really? You're going to bother a whole-ass stranger in the middle of the day because you think they're physically attractive? How would you feel if that happened to you while you had somewhere to be? Please find other socially acceptable places to initiate conversations with strangers…and only do so as if you're talking to a complete stranger, regardless of whether they're physically attractive or not. Do this because they're a complete fucking stranger and you're probably not attractive to them or compatible with them long-term in the first place. And no, that's not negative thinking…it's just reality.

If it feels daunting to talk to someone attractive, get back to fucking basics. Recall how you talked to people back in elementary school at the lunch table. Remember how you would find someone with a similar type of backpack or shirt that you own, or maybe just make a random observation about the environment you are both in and strike up a convo about it. It's not that hard, I promise. And stop doing things solely to impress other people—do things for you, and out of your own curiosity or desire, if you will. It's amazing how this leads to authentic interactions. You can also have an opinion that someone is physically attractive and not have a romantic connection with them. Common fucking sense for the win.

While I'm at it, let's add in some more common sense. If something is being done to you by another person that feels mean or wrong, trust your gut. A good indicator for this is if it's something you wouldn't do to someone you cared about, like a close family member or friend—that's a good indication that something weird is going on. Treat the conflict in these situations the same way you would with any of them. Please don't overcomplicate this because of an outcome bias. Let the facts of the situation and their reflective character do the talking. We'll soon get into how to taper any overemotional investment that complicates these situations.

It goes without saying, but **stop listening to dating advice** unless you're learning to identify other people who use it. In studying for this book, I recall reading a certain scumbag's book on seduction and having my stomach turn knowing that a certain ex-girlfriend of mine had unknowingly used several of these tactics on me. Thankfully, no matter how much a person tries to cover it up, a piece of shit eventually just ends up smelling and looking like one. Fast forward to today, and I actually feel sorry for people like her and those who use this shitty advice. It's unfortunate, but they always get what's coming to them.

Now that's done, let's discuss moving forward, indirectly, of course. Most single daters end up at the following fork in the road—this being an exception, with three options instead of two:

1) Accept your current marketplace capabilities and date one of your available options.

2) Self-improve and/or looks max. This road takes you on a journey that will loop you back into the same marketplace to reassess your options.

3) Do nothing different, stay stagnant at the fork in the road, and don't change anything at all. And then die alone, several years younger than you would have otherwise, with most likely a less fulfilled life.

I think you can infer which option this book recommends, but I digress. The choice is always yours.

The next point I'll make is around the science of new love and making your emotional investment iterative correlating to the amount of time you've known them. In my first book *From Brokenhearted to Brave,* I talk about the six-month chemical high. In a study conducted by scientific researchers, new couples had their dopamine and serotonin levels measured during the initial phases of a new relationship. For the first six months, these levels were elevated from their normal baseline due to the euphoria that falling-in-love sensations create. These heightened levels took six months (yes, six months) to fully clear before they returned to normal. [27] Understanding this is paramount when

---

entering new relationships. I will have hacks at the end of the chapter to show how you can reduce this six-month period, too, and focus on what's really important from a long-term perspective.

The last points I will make are around all the other areas I didn't touch on. I know that several other factors have also contributed to this widespread singlehood crisis: changes in marriage and family law, the rise of social media, the decline of religious values, economic challenges faced by generations younger than the baby boomers, overt societal support for singles via various businesses, housing shortages, and the harmful effects of pornography. I'm sure I missed a few, too. I choose to focus on the specific challenges I see with people who post about them on social media, as they appear to genuinely care. If this chapter is popular, I might dedicate an entire book to breaking down the rest of these factors, along with getting truly specific on toxic dating movements. Anyone who lies, overgeneralizes, or overemphasizes bullshit "facts" and tries to take advantage of people and their singlehood can get it. It might just be too easy for me, though. I'm already disinterested at the thought. And, I kind of hated writing most of this chapter. Nobody likes eating pieces of shit for breakfast, unless their name is Shooter McGavin…baby. Hey, anytime you can work in a Happy Gilmore reference, you should do it, amirite? The leaders of these so-called dating advice movements are nothing more than Shooter McGavin's themselves—morons, douchebags, and haters all wrapped into one! Insert a "You don't want the smoke, move along" GIF here.

IN SUMMARY:

- Understand the science of physical attraction, have realistic expectations and emphasize dating someone with relative dating marketplace value, as it's the best foundation for romantic relationships. Choose the fork in the road analogy option that best suits you and your longer-term dating goals. Then, prioritize said longer term criteria.

- Stop using for-pay dating apps that are financially incentivized to keep you single. Instead, utilize free options like Facebook Dating, free Facebook and other online dating groups that schedule in-person events, and meetup apps. Save your money and time and avoid these awful and ineffective businesses.

- Stop listening to all direct dating advice. These people will only lead you to short-term results and long-term hell. Unfollow anyone who solicits this advice on social media, unless you're learning to actively avoid people who use it.

- You can think that someone is physically attractive and not have a romantic connection with them. Get back to basics with your conversational skills and stop overemphasizing someone's physical attraction. Also, deal with conflict the way you would with anyone else close to you. Learn to be yourself and act authentically, regardless of romantic interest.

Then, work on anything you have weaknesses in, essentially removing the dating element from the context.

- While nothing is guaranteed in life, people vastly underestimate how much marriage and monogamy actually protects each other. Learn to manage the potential downfalls if you're concerned about divorce with prenuptial agreements and counseling, etc. Take your time and choose long term partners as wisely as you can.

- Here are dating hacks to look past the six-month chemical high:

  - Make sure you have high standards when it comes to value system alignment, personality, morals, and character, and put less emphasis on butterfly feelings.

  - Partners eventually become the closest of family. Pay close attention to how they treat and talk about their closest family. (I can't emphasize this one enough!) Check in with yourself to see if you get any icks and address them with your partner.

  - Ask them to name five things they like about themselves and three things they find difficult about themselves or think others might struggle with when dealing with them. If they say there is nothing difficult about them and they like everything, this is the reddest of flags. Conversely, if they don't like anything about themselves, this is a glaring red flag, too.

- For more dating questions, you can check out the book *101 Questions to Ask Before You Get Engaged* by H. Norman Wright[28] and review, modify as necessary, and mix in a few questions based on the level of importance to you. There are also tips for additional red flags to watch out for in their recommendations in the book, and the PDF version is available free online with a Google search.

As you can see, I care a lot about all of this. I hope this info and guidance help you for real because these are the things I wish I knew years ago. If you feel like dating is hard, you're not alone. I used to be right there with you. But don't worry, things get so much better after working to find the real you. And more good news is that the end of the book is in sight, too!

Chapter Thirteen: Beneath the Surface

I choose this chapter name because 'things aren't always as they appear' quotes are kinda lame, and you already know how I feel about the overuse of quotes in books. Partner that with the fact the last chapter felt really long, and I typically like shorter chapters with more condensed points. I'm getting back to my roots here. This book would not be complete without this last-minute add, though. The fact of the matter is, the solutions to some of my biggest problems—ones that took the longest to solve—came from issues that seemed totally unrelated. I'm typically a pretty logical person. But sometimes, appearance logic is the enemy, and what's beneath the surface is what matters. I guess you could say problem solving is also like a box of chocolates…You really never do know what you're going to get! That is, unless you read the labels. If only there were labels for solving problems…cue this book for some, though!

Much like addition by subtraction in Chapter Four, the increase of salt being the key to solving my staph and improving my skin issues in Chapter Five, or the posture exercises being the catalyst to fully unlocking the hinge on my jaw in Chapter Ten, in the next story I am about to tell, the answers to so many of our problems within our bodies are tricky. It's the real reason we need to continue to improve in all ways. To really listen to our bodies. Then, to tinker. You never know when another small improvement may be the answer to a huge nagging problem.

For years, I have struggled on and off with not-so-white teeth. And until lately, it was never anything egregious. I personally think that super white teeth look unnatural, so I never really chased it. But for the last year or so, my teeth were particularly bad. I tried a few all-natural whitening toothpaste ideas with no luck. When I asked my dentist, she said that I hardly had any enamel left. She said not to try any additional whitening products as they wouldn't work and that I was getting down to the base layer of my teeth, which is naturally yellow. Since I was planning on getting braces, she recommended that I may want to get veneers. Given that I can be stubborn as hell with issues like this, I'm sure you know what's coming up next. I ventured off to find my own solution!

When I researched in holistic dentistry, I found one who said that everything we need to rebuild our enamel is in our saliva. Supposedly, our saliva can remineralize our teeth if we let our teeth sit in it every day for several months, especially in the afternoon. After a few months of this, nothing improved. My simple mind then thought, *what's been the wonder mineral for me*? Salt. I had already ditched my traditional store-bought toothpaste for an all-natural formula years ago because it massively aggravated my autoimmune issues, and I experienced decent results. Plus, after I had the thought, I had read in some comments on other tooth-whitening videos on YouTube of people doing this, too, so I thought, *Let's give it a try.* So, before bed, I began brushing my teeth with some water and a few grains of coarse kosher salt. To enhance the process, I also cut out all sweet citrus from my diet and replaced it with vitamin water and lemon water to hit my every-other-day vitamin C target. Although my mouth felt way cleaner and I have never experienced bleeding gums after this, there was still not much difference in the whiteness after a few months.

I'm sure you can tell what's coming next—enter what appeared to be a totally unrelated issue. After my kidney donation surgery, as part of the kidney clinic I was referred to, they informed me that I was low in vitamin D and that it was a key supplement for me to take. For years, I had done so with no issues, and I also made it a point to get out in the sun more in the warmer months. But, since switching to a more MTHFR-based diet a few years ago, I still took the supplement at the same dose during the low UV index months. Instead of taking 2,000 IUs a day, I took 4,000 IUs every other day because my stomach didn't jive with it on a daily basis—and it seemed to interact negatively with the marijuana edibles I took every other day. Then, this winter, I began noticing some strange issues. My lymph nodes were still pretty swollen, even without the presence of other autoimmune issues. I noticed some other things, along with my teeth appearing even darker than normal. I was starting to become concerned.

The vitamin D was the only supplement I was taking, and I was eating various greens to get my corresponding vitamin K2. I started reading up on signs that I was taking too much and found several that were leading to potential vitamin D toxicity. Even though I hadn't altered my dose, I believe this probably occurred because of my improvements in my gut's nutrient absorption once I was on an optimal diet. So, I stopped taking the supplement approximately a month ago. I almost immediately began feeling better in multiple ways. All the aforementioned symptoms had subsided, and the funniest thing happened: My teeth appeared much less dark.

I was perplexed, so I started researching again. Supposedly, when you take too much vitamin D, it can cause over-calcification in the blood or, in simpler terms, too much calcium. That calcification can cause your teeth to darken. Wild. I sit here today with visibly whiter teeth than they were a few weeks ago. And even though they aren't fully white, I even got complimented on them the other day! Due to my age, I know that some yellowing is normal, but once I get my braces off in a few months, I'll test enhancing my efforts with other solutions I saw, like ground cloves and coconut oil, etc. And if I ever experience any vitamin D deficiencies again, I'll add back in a much smaller dose.

After this happened, I wanted to see if there was any way I could have noticed this ahead of time by searching for the root cause in reverse. I searched 'indirect causes of yellow teeth' on Google and their Gemini AI, but nothing mentioned calcification. Had I just focused on the symptom of the yellow teeth, I would have never known. But if you search for 'Does calcification cause yellow teeth?', it comes right up and confirms it.[29] This is why I believe we always need to strive to optimize our supplement and diet protocols. So many things impact other things. Since this was absolutely one of my most frustrating problems to improve upon, I'm glad I made some progress in time to include it in this book!

IN SUMMARY:

- Always think outside of the box when approaching issues and continue improving. You never know when improving a seemingly unrelated issue can drastically positively impact other problems.

- Keep an open mind, and look at things beneath the surface when tackling a seemingly really difficult and stubborn problem, as its solution is probably multifaceted.

I just love solving tough problems, don't you? And I'm excited to see my dentist again and tell her what happened, as she's also a long-time family friend. We'll see what she says about my enamel, too. Gosh, I am such a nerd for this self-improvement stuff, but I can't help myself! I'm also excited that the next chapter is also the last before the conclusion. Let's start putting a bow on finishing this book!

Chapter Fourteen: The Reality of Glowing Up

Much like the daring to compare chapter, I need to wrap up the book by spending some time on my not-so-positive or expected experiences since getting to know the real me. I will caveat the following statements and research with the fact that overall, it's still a huge benefit, and I'd never go back. I just wish I was prepared for some of the things that have happened post-glow-up. Glowing up has advantages and disadvantages. It can bring up other insecurities, especially if you're an introvert deep down like me. Being aware of them is key. External validation can also be dangerous and treacherous. Your personal values can and will probably be tested once you start experiencing results. Finally, honing your newfound glow with other semi-related refinements to optimize everything can be fun, too.

Let's start with some interesting research from the land of neuroscience. Do you know that awkward feeling when you make eye contact with someone you're looking at or catch looking at you? If you're anything like me, you immediately look away, right? Yeah. I recently learned that this looking away is triggering a process in your brain called self-referential processing. Don't worry—I had no idea what that meant either. In simpler terms, in these situations when someone makes eye contact with you, what you think about yourself is what you'll convey. If you're not confident in yourself, it causes you to react in this way. That's definitely telling. I will wait until the end of the chapter to discuss how I tackled this and to end on a positive note.

Now, let's talk about the not-so-positive notes. There were many unexpected challenges I have encountered since glowing up. As you can see from the dating rant chapter, I had to completely relearn how to date. I had to learn how my changes impacted what others thought of me. When you become more desirable, you must stay keenly aware of an individual's true nature and intent. People around you also begin to not shoot you straight more often. Because they either don't want you to change or maybe care more about what you think since you're different now, they oftentimes just tell you what they think you want to hear. One thing's for sure—self-improvements cause other indirectly related changes you wouldn't expect for sure.

But the most surprising ones left me with some very unexpected despair. You see, I thought that these good-looking, seemingly "happy" couples were exactly that: happy. Try telling that to some of these wives out there. I just assumed that since people were good-looking and had what a lot of us single people wanted, they were content. Boy, was I wrong. Without going into too much detail, since my glow-up, I have had several beautiful married women try to get in contact with me. Some have even tried to cross lines. Women who otherwise wanted nothing to do with me back in the day had since taken a newfound interest in me. Imagine that. Coincidence? I think not. Some of my family members and I have also noticed several married women repetitively making eye contact or all-out staring at me in public…most when they're with their husbands! It freaks me out. Not everyone acts like this, obviously, but I was very naïve to the ones that did. It really shocked me. As someone who wants to get remarried someday, it has messed with my psyche quite a bit. Expecting these situations and making sure you're prepared for them will make them easier to handle.

Going back to conveying what you think about yourself, I want to touch on my last point. Things like your style may need to be addressed, even after your glow-up work, to help improve this. I enjoy taking some pride in my fashion and looking presentable, but I don't spend much money on it. I recommend form-fitting clothes and not spending a lot of money on name brands unless you want to attract people who value that, too. In my humble opinion, you should be the star, not what you wear. Your hairstyle does matter some, too, and facial hair can be a game-changer for men, one way or another. Optimizing it based on what you like is key. Once you feel good about and like what you see in yourself, your self-referential processing goes down along with your false self-beliefs, and others will feel that, too. Heck, you might even hold that gaze at an attractive, non-married person and smile, too! Have fun with some of this, too, once you've earned it.

IN SUMMARY:

- Books have covers to judge and words to read for a reason. Don't fall in love with the façade of the exposed. Look beneath the surface with people, too. You might be surprised by what you find.

- Instead of abruptly looking away after making eye contact with someone, try offering a smile and holding their gaze briefly before turning your attention elsewhere.

- Beware of certain perceived 'benefits.' You'll have to pass on a lot of bad and avoid a lot of pitfalls to find the good and where you are supposed to be in life.

Epilogue

As I come to the end of writing this book, it oddly culminates with other major life events right around the corner. My youngest of two kiddos will be graduating from high school and going off to college in a matter of days, and I plan on selling our family home to move halfway across the country to further pursue my dreams. Now that I know the real me, I have all new dreams, new ambitions, and a much greater appreciation for life. I know if I can do it, anyone can. Never forget how strong you are, too. How do I know you're strong? You're still breathing. And as long as that's the case, you can always persevere and achieve the realistic and even not-so-realistic goals you set for yourself along the way.

I now leave you with an understanding of how the science behind the intertwinement of various improvements can create a cyclical impact across all areas of your life. It's the most important lesson in this book. If you take only one thing from it, let it be that. When I reflect on this journey, it's tough to say what one thing made me improve the most; in reality, it was a combination of all these things and the wisdom gained from the experiences as a whole. This info came into your life for a reason, so use it and make it better. Remember to show yourself love. Real love. And prove it with your actions for YOU. Once you do this and the end result is the best you can do, it grants you acceptance of the conclusion and gives you a genuine path forward. What an immense blessing, to say the least.

No matter what my take was on "glowing up", you will certainly have your own personalized experiences as well. I view myself in this position to be a tour guide on an elaborate hike to a beautiful waterfall. I may be able to guide you there, but I cannot tell you how to feel about it once you arrive. And once you follow much of this advice, you will *arrive.* Also, I will refence a relative stock market analogy to showcase how I feel about my newfound self now. They don't let you buy stock for cheaper after it's worth more now just because you owned it in the past. I don't let people who sold my metaphorical stock when the price was low to buy me back at the same price now that the value is worth far more. Remember that, if you'd like, for after you complete your journey, too. Your growth is yours, nobody else's. Only you get to decide what you do with it.

I wouldn't be able to learn as much as I have unless the smart people around me shared what they knew. A huge thanks goes out to all the doctors, authors, and health practitioners who helped me on this journey. And saving the best for last, you, the reader! None of this is possible without you, so thanks hardly covers it. I hope you can sense the smile I have thinking about your journey through my words. The fact that you care about self-improvement enough to read a book like this makes us kindred spirits, at least in my book. And this is…my book. *Ugh*, I've tried, but I don't think I can ever give dad jokes up. Just kidding, I would never do that!

Lastly, remember the only real thing that will improve your dating situation—or any other challenging situation in life for that matter—is genuinely improving all of who you are, for YOU. As you grow, be aware of all the changes around you, as there will be many. Oh, and don't forget to enjoy it! We all get to write our own stories. As an author, I can only hope that mine will help yours. I've gone through a lot of struggles, some of my own making for sure and some definitely not. But, after everything I've accomplished, I'm happy with how God made me. God made you a certain way for a reason, too! Embrace all that comes with it, and you'll be amazed by the real YOU.

Well, that's it for me for now. If you want to continue keeping up with me, you can follow me on all the main socials @Thoroughwayne. Continue to take good care of yourself—you are the most qualified. Until next time!

Bibliography

1. Wayne, J. (n.d.). *Courage is being scared to death but saddling up anyway* [Quote]. Goodreads. https://www.goodreads.com/quotes/13533-courage-is-being-scared-to-death-but-saddling-up-anyway

2. Einstein, A. (n.d.). *The measure of intelligence is the ability to change.* Goodreads. https://www.goodreads.com/quotes/85475-the-measure-of-intelligence-is-the-ability-to-change

3. Bryant, K. (n.d.). *The measure of intelligence is the ability to change.* TikTok. https://www.tiktok.com/@motivative.minds/video/7195331429738335493

4. Google. (2025, February 14). *[AI-generated response to the prompt "What's more important: diet or exercise?"].* Gemini. https://www.google.com

5. Google. (2025, February 14). *[AI-generated response to the prompt "How many people have the MTHFR gene mutation?"].* Gemini. https://www.google.com

6. The Diary of a CEO Clips (2024). *These products are secretly making you & your future kids sick.... | No.1 toxicologist [YouTube video].* YouTube. https://www.youtube.com/watch?v=joG8JdhZyoM

7. The Diary of a CEO Clips (2024). *The most toxic kitchen items slowly killing you... | No.1 toxicologist Dr.*

Yvonne Burkart [YouTube video]. YouTube. https://www.youtube.com/watch?v=q1Qpv0gHnTc

8. The Diary of a CEO Clips (2024). *The most toxic kitchen items slowly killing you... | No.1 toxicologist Dr. Yvonne Burkart [YouTube video].* YouTube. https://www.youtube.com/watch?v=q1Qpv0gHnTc

9. Microsoft. (2025, February 14). *[Search result for "What risks do genetically modified foods cause?"].* Bing. https://www.bing.com

10. Google. (2025, February 14). *[AI-generated response to the prompt "Sugar and salt, specifically glucose and sodium, play crucial roles in hydration by aiding in the absorption and retention of water in the body."].* Gemini. https://www.google.com

11. Google. (2025, February 14). *[AI-generated response to the prompt "How much salt and glucose per glass of water?"].* Gemini. https://www.google.com

12. Google. (2025, February 14). *[AI-generated response to the prompt "FDA daily sodium recommendation."].* Gemini. https://www.google.com

13. DiNicolantonio, J. (2017). *The salt fix.* Dreamscape Media. https://www.audible.com/pd/The-Salt-Fix-Audiobook/

14. Fuller, T. (n.d.). *Health is not valued until sickness comes*. BrainyQuote. https://www.brainyquote.com/quotes/thomas_fuller_380713

15. Gottfried, S. S. (2024). *The autoimmune cure.* HarperCollins Publishers. https://www.audible.com/pd/The-Autoimmune-Cure-Audiobook/

16. Google. (2025, February 14). *[AI-generated response to the prompt "What are epigenetics?"].* Gemini. https://www.google.com

17. Google. (2025, February 14). *[AI-generated response to the prompt "Four main epigenetic mechanisms."].* Gemini. https://www.google.com

18. McGarey, G. (2024). *The well-lived life.* Simon & Schuster. https://www.audible.com/pd/The-Well-Lived-Life-Audiobook/

19. Google. (2025, February 14). *[AI-generated response to the prompt "What percentage of a person's physical attraction is based on your face?"].* Gemini. https://www.google.com

20. Wikipedia (2024). *Facial symmetry.* Wikipedia. https://en.wikipedia.org/wiki/Facial_symmetry

21. Wikipedia (2025). *Averageness.* Wikipedia. https://en.wikipedia.org/wiki/Averageness

22. Hopkins Medicine (2025). *Hemifacial microsomia.* Johns Hopkins Medicine. https://www.hopkinsmedicine.org/health/conditions-and-diseases/cleft-lip-and-palate/hemifacial-microsomia

23. Google. (2025, February 14). *[AI-generated response to the prompt "Facial Torsion"].* Gemini. https://www.google.com.

24. Google. (2025, February 14). *[AI-generated response to the prompt "What percentage of 40-year-olds are not married?"]*. Gemini. https://www.google.com

25. Google. (2025, February 14). *[AI-generated response to the prompt "How many people in the US between the ages of 40–49?"]*. Gemini. https://www.google.com

26. TLC (2025). *The science of attraction*. The Learning Channel. https://www.tlc.com/

27. Psych2Go. "The 8 Stages of Dating." YouTube video. Last modified January 5, 2020. https://www.youtube.com/watch?v=X6Hk7hIAStw

28. Wright, H. N. (2004). *101 questions to ask before you get engaged.* Harvest House Publishers. https://www.amazon.com/101-Questions-Ask-Before-Engaged/

29. Google. (2025, February 14). *[AI-generated response to the prompt "Does calcification cause yellow teeth?"]*. Gemini. https://www.google.com

Made in the USA
Monee, IL
11 November 2026

51388003-e91e-48a2-a23e-3e48e76119d4R02